COOKBOOK FOR PARKINSON'S DISEASE

A Perfect Parkinson's Disease Diet: What To Eat And Avoid

KADIE PLUMLEY

Table of Contents

CHAPTER ONE

Diet for Parkinson's Disease

Parkinson's Disease Diet: What to Eat and Avoid

If you have Parkinson's disease, you don't need to adhere to a specific diet. You may be unable to properly nourish yourself if you suffer from a condition that makes it difficult to move your body. To maintain your strength and keep your Parkinson's meds working as they should, you'll need to eat a diet rich in vitamins and minerals.

For Parkinson's sufferers, it's common to experience weight loss, difficulty swallowing and pooping, and nausea from medication. Your physician or a licensed dietitian may be able to help you figure out the best course of action to take in dealing with those problems.

Eating a Healthy Diet

Make sure to eat a wide variety of foods from each food group.

Check with your doctor first if you think you need vitamin supplements.

Maintaining a healthy weight for your height and age can be accomplished through regular exercise and a well-balanced diet.

Fiber-rich foods like broccoli, peas, apples, cooked split peas and beans, whole-grain breads, cereals, and pasta should be a regular part of your diet.

Reduce your intake of added sugar, salt, and saturated fats

from animal products like meat and dairy products, as well as high cholesterol.

You should drink at least eight cups of water each day.

Consult your physician to determine whether or not you are permitted to consume alcoholic beverages. It may interfere with the proper functioning of your medications.

Medication and Food Co-Administration

Parkinson's disease patients should take levodopa. On an empty stomach or at least one hour after a meal, it is recommended that you take it. However, some people may feel queasy as a result of this. Your doctor may prescribe a different medication or a different combination of medications, and this may or may not alleviate your nausea. If this is the case, your physician may advise you to take medication to alleviate your symptoms.

Ask your doctor if cutting back on protein is necessary. A high-protein diet may impair the effectiveness of levodopa in some patients.

Getting Rid of the Morning Sickness

Drinks that are clear or icy cold are best. Sugary drinks may be more effective at calming your stomach than water.

Keep away from orange and grapefruit juices and other acidic drinks.

Slowly savor each sip.

Instead of consuming liquids during meals, drink them between them.

Have saltine crackers or plain bread for a meal that isn't spicy or flavorful.
Avoid foods that are fried, greasy, or sugary in any way..

Slowly savor each mouthful and eat more frequently.

Make sure you don't eat hot and cold foods at the same time.

Avoid nausea caused by the smell of hot or warm foods by eating cold or room-temperature meals.

After a meal, take a few minutes to relax, but keep your head up. Getting your heart rate up and moving around can make nausea worse and even cause you to vomit.

Brushing your teeth after a meal is a bad idea.

Having a few crackers before getting out of bed can help ease nausea. A high-protein snack, such as lean meats or cheese, is a good idea before going to bed.

Eat when you're not feeling so sick.

Drinking or Mouth Dryness
The side effects of some Parkinson's medications can include dehydration. There are a number of things you can do to alleviate your pain

CHAPTER TWO

Make an effort to get your recommended daily fluid intake of 8 cups up to this point. The fluid levels of some Parkinson's sufferers may need to be monitored. Ask your doctor how much water you should be drinking.

Reduce the amount of caffeine in your diet by limiting your intake of caffeine-rich beverages like coffee, tea, cola and chocolate.

Breads, toast, cookies, and crackers can be softened by

putting them in the microwave for a few seconds. When you're done, you can slurp them up with milk or decaf tea or coffee.

Each time you take a bite of food, sip a sip of water to help you swallow.

Adding sauces to food will soften and moisten it, thus making it more enjoyable. Cooking with butter is a great option.

To increase saliva production and moisten your mouth, try eating sour candy or fruit ice.

Most mouthwashes contain alcohol, which can dry out your mouth, so avoid them. Find out if there is anything else you can do from your doctor or dentist.

Obtain prescription artificial saliva from your doctor.

Making the Decision to Eat When You're Exhausted

In the event that you find yourself unable to eat at a later time in the day, you can:

Save your energy for eating by preparing simple foods. If you live with your family, let them help you prepare your meal.

Consider using a courier service. They're available in some supermarkets. You can also see if your local Meals on Wheels program will deliver food to you for free or for a small fee.

Keep fresh fruits and vegetables and high-fiber cold cereals on hand for healthy snacks.

Make extra food and store it in the freezer for quick meals when you're feeling under the weather.

Enjoy your meal by getting plenty of rest prior to sitting down to eat. Eat your largest meal of the day first thing in the morning to give your body the energy it needs for the rest of the day.

When You're Hungry But Not Hungry Enough

You may not want to eat at all on some days.

Your doctor can help you. Depression can lead to a lack of appetite. When you receive treatment, you can expect your appetite to return.

Make yourself hungry by taking a walk or engaging in some other light activity.

After you've finished your meal, drink a beverage so that you don't feel full before the next one.

Make sure to include your favorite foods on the menu. Begin by devouring the most calorific foods on your plate. Avoid sugary sodas, candy, and chips, however.

Mix things up by trying new foods and ingredients.

Snacks with a high amount of protein and calories, such as

• Dessert: ice cream.

• Cheese

• Bars of granola

• Custard

• Sandwiches

With cheese, nachos are even better.

• Eggs

• Peanut butter-covered crackers

Half-and-Half Cereal

• Yogurt made with greek yogurt

Maintain a Proper Body Mass Index

People with Parkinson's are more prone to malnutrition and

weight loss than the general population. So, keeping tabs on your weight is a smart idea.

Unless your doctor advises you to weigh yourself more frequently, weigh yourself no more than once or twice per week. When taking diuretics or steroids like prednisone, you should weigh yourself every day to monitor your weight loss.

Consult your physician if you noticeably gain or lose weight (2 pounds in a day or 5 pounds in a week). They may want to alter your diet in order to treat your illness.

If you want to put on weight, follow these steps:

Consult your physician to determine whether or not nutritional supplements are appropriate for you. A few of them can be dangerous or interfere with your medication.

Avoid low-fat or low-calorie foods unless you've been specifically instructed to do so. Make your own yogurt and cheese by using whole milk

CHAPTER THREE

Parkinson's Disease Dietary Recommendations: What to Eat and How Nutrition Can Help

When it comes to managing Parkinson's disease, food is an essential part of overall health and wellness. Eating a well-balanced diet can be difficult if you have symptoms like nausea, swallowing problems, or even tremors, but it is critical if you have any of these.

According to the Parkinson's Foundation, a healthy diet helps your prescription medications work optimally, keeps your bones strong, combats constipation and weight loss, and helps maintain your physical health.

For Indu Subramanian, MD, a UCLA neurology specialist in wellness and integrative medicine, the use of diet and nutrition is not a substitute for medication but rather complements it. Regardless of whether or not you have Parkinson's disease, a healthy lifestyle, including a well-balanced diet, is beneficial.

Changes in eating habits due to Parkinson's disease

It is possible to notice changes in your appetite and eating habits if you have been diagnosed with Parkinson's disease, says Dr. Subramanian.

Many prescription medications may work better on an empty stomach, but they may also cause nausea in some people.

If at all possible, Subramanian says, patients should take their medication about an hour before meals in order to avoid protein interactions. The body's ability to process some Parkinson's disease medications can be hampered if protein-rich foods such as meat, fish, eggs, dairy, nuts, and beans are consumed too close to the time of medication administration.

Your doctor may advise you to eat a small snack like crackers or applesauce before taking your medication if you get nauseated after taking it on an empty stomach.

Subramanian also points out that Parkinson's disease sufferers are concerned about losing weight due to a loss of appetite. Eating can be made difficult by symptoms such as trouble swallowing, a decreased capacity for tasting and smelling, nausea associated with medication use, and movement problems (in the hands and wrists).

Use of rubber mats to keep dishes from slipping while being consumed

• Using a "Parkinson's spoon" or other weighted utensils and cups

Avoiding spills by using a cup with a lid or straw

In order to make it easier to swallow, cut food into smaller pieces and chew thoroughly before swallowing eating soups and pureed dishes

Consuming bitter green vegetables like kale or spinach, as well as spicy foods, to stimulate your appetite and enhance the flavor of your meals.

• Increasing hunger by exercising just before a meal

When Eating and Drinking is Difficult, a "Parkinson's Spoon" Can Help.

Certain foods may be difficult to eat if you have Parkinson's disease symptoms like tremor, stiff joints, or difficulty swallowing. In order to make eating and drinking easier, Subramanian recommends consulting an occupational therapist.

A "Parkinson's spoon" is one option. People with Parkinson's disease will appreciate the convenience of using this well-liked gadget during mealtime. Products vary, but they're all eating utensils that have been fitted with a design or technology that makes them more stable while you eat..

Psychologists, speech pathologists, and dietitians can all provide assistance.

Talking to a registered dietitian can help you make changes to your diet, such as learning how to thicken liquids or soften solid foods.

Speech-language pathologists may be able to help if swallowing remains a problem for you in the future.

In order to conduct a swallow study, a speech pathologist who also works as a swallow therapist can conduct a test in which you eat a variety of foods and the X-ray machine is used to monitor your swallowing, says Subramanian. It is possible for Parkinson's disease sufferers to experience food aspiration, which occurs when food enters the lungs, so your doctor may recommend a swallow study to identify problem foods.

Finally, because anxiety and depression are common in Parkinson's patients and can lead to a loss of appetite, it's important to be aware of these symptoms and seek treatment if necessary.

What Are the Healthiest Foods to Consume if You Have Parkinson's?

Most people with Parkinson's don't need to drastically alter their eating habits if they were eating well before getting the diagnosis in the first place. Some additional considerations should be taken into account.

CHAPTER FOUR

The Parkinson's Foundation recommends a diet rich in grains like brown rice and breads, vegetables, fruits, and lean protein such as beans. As a group, these foods provide a wide range of nutrients to help you maintain a healthy weight while providing your body with the essential nutrients it needs.

In Parkinson's disease, "the Mediterranean Diet has become popular," says Subramanian. "We recommend it to many of our patients." In addition, we recommend the Mind Diet, which is low in salt and aimed at enhancing brain function. Processed foods and foods with artificial or simple sugars should be avoided whenever possible. Eat as many whole foods and plant-based diets as you can."

Maintaining a healthy weight by eating in accordance with the MyPlate recommendations of the United States Department of Agriculture (USDA) is another benefit of adhering to the USDA's MyPlate diet guidelines. If you have Parkinson's disease, you may want to eat more calcium, magnesium, and vitamin D and K-rich foods in your diet to keep your bones strong.

Bone-building nutrients can be found in a variety of foods, including:

• Salmon

• Milk

• Eggs

• Spinach

Several types of nuts, such as almonds

In addition, because vitamin D deficiency is common in Parkinson's disease patients, Subramanian recommends speaking with your doctor about whether you should increase your intake of the important nutrient for bone and gut health (and perhaps brain health as well). Aside from fortified dairy products, she recommends eating eggs, egg yolks, and fatty fish like salmon for getting adequate amounts of vitamin D, too.

Exactly How Do Antioxidant-Rich Foods Benefit Parkinson's Disease?

Free radicals are potentially harmful molecules that our bodies produce, and antioxidants help fight them. According to the Parkinson's Foundation, some researchers believe that oxidative stress, or nerve cell damage, caused by free radicals may be linked to Parkinson's disease. However, antioxidant supplements have not been shown to be effective in treating Parkinson's disease, according to the organization.

Subramanian recommends eating a diet rich in antioxidants, such as brightly colored and dark fruits like berries and leafy green vegetables. In addition, certain nuts, according to her, have been linked to better brain health.

These are some of the most antioxidant-rich foods, according to a landmark study published in Nutrition Journal in 2010 that cataloged more than 3,000 food items.

• Apples that have been dipped in apple juice.

• Blackberries

• Apricots

• Artichokes

The dried fruit of the mango

• Raspberries

Plums that have been dried

• Strawberries

Is Parkinson's Helped by Drinking Green Tea?

According to a review published in March 2016 in the journal CNS Neurological Disorders-Drug Targets, some studies have found that green tea, which is also high in antioxidants, can slow the progression of Parkinson's disease and other neurodegenerative disorders. To date, no one has figured out exactly how green tea works to prevent these ailments, or even how much of it is safe and effective.

Parkinson's Disease: Constipation and Hydration

The Parkinson's Foundation recommends a daily fiber intake of 20 to 25 grams in order to maintain bowel health, as Parkinson's disease can cause constipation.

Maintaining a regular bowel movement is critical for overall health, according to Subramanian. "As much vegetables and fiber as your body can handle is what we recommend," say the researchers. In addition, foods rich in prebiotics, like sauerkraut and kimchee, can be beneficial."

You should check with your doctor before incorporating fermented foods into your diet because some Parkinson's disease medications don't work as well when they're paired with fermented foods.

Everyone, including those with Parkinson's disease, should drink plenty of water to stay hydrated. The Parkinson's Foundation recommends drinking six to eight glasses of water a day and taking your medication with a full glass of water. It may help your body better break down the medication.

Constipation and high blood pressure can both be helped by regular hydration, as Subramanian explains. For Parkinson's patients, we recommend drinking 40 ounces of water per day. There's no coffee, tea, or anything else in there. Improved digestion is another possible benefit of this."

Try celery, butternut squash, grapefruit, strawberries, and

watermelon instead of drinking water if it causes you to feel nauseous.

Dietary Restrictions for People with Parkinson's Disease

Some of the same foods that can harm people without Parkinson's disease should be avoided by people with the disease in order to maintain good health.

A high-sugar diet, for example, may cause you to overindulge in calories while also depriving your body of essential nutrients. Dental decay and diabetes are also linked to it.

Sodium-rich foods can also raise blood pressure and increase the risk of heart attack and stroke. Foods that are high in salt, according to the American Heart Association, include:

• Rolls and loaves of bread

• Pizza

• Sandwiches

• Cured meats and cold cuts

- Soup

- Tacos and burritos

Due to the dysfunction of the autonomic nervous system in Parkinson's disease, most of our patients experience low blood pressure," says Subramanian. If you're experiencing low blood pressure, you may benefit from a little extra salt in your diet or even energy drinks.

When it comes to managing your blood pressure and Parkinson's disease, you should consult with your doctor before making any changes to your diet.

It's also a good idea to avoid foods that are high in calories and saturated or trans fat, which can raise your risk of heart disease, cancer, and weight gain.

If you have Parkinson's disease and find it difficult to get out and about, it's critical that you keep track of how many calories you're taking in and how much exercise you're getting.

Alcoholic beverages, on the other hand, contribute a significant amount of calories while providing your body with little to no nutritional value. In addition, drinking alcohol can increase the likelihood of a fall or other accident. If you're going to drink, talk to your doctor first to see if there are any possible interactions between your medication and alcohol.

THE END